The Superfood Revolution

Nutrients to Transform Your Life

Table of Contents

1. Introduction 1

2. Understanding Superfoods: The Basics 2

    2.1. Understanding the Superfood Concept 2

    2.2. Nutritional Density: A Key Aspect 3

    2.3. Superfoods: More than Vitamins and Minerals 3

    2.4. Staying Grounded: The 'Super' Misconception 4

    2.5. Embracing the Superfood Journey 4

3. The Antioxidant Army: Superfoods for Immunity 6

    3.1. Understanding Antioxidants 6

    3.2. The Superfood Squadron 6

        3.2.1. Berries 7

        3.2.2. Nuts and Seeds 7

        3.2.3. Herbs and Spices 7

        3.2.4. Leafy Greens 7

    3.3. Empower Your Diet with Antioxidant-rich Superfoods 8

        3.3.1. Incorporate Berries into Your Meals 8

        3.3.2. Pair Your Meals with Nuts and Seeds 8

        3.3.3. Get Creative with Herbs and Spices 8

        3.3.4. Regularly Consume Leafy Greens 8

    3.4. Beware of Excess 8

4. Brain Power: Superfoods for Cognitive Function 10

    4.1. Understanding the Brain-Food Connection 10

    4.2. 1. Berries 10

    4.3. 2. Fatty Fish 11

    4.4. 3. Dark Chocolate 11

    4.5. 4. Green Tea 11

    4.6. 5. Turmeric 12

    4.7. 6. Broccoli 12

4.8. 7. Pumpkin Seeds ... 12

4.9. Implementing Superfoods into Your Diet ... 12

4.10. A Word of Caution ... 13

5. Weight Warriors: Superfoods for Weight Management ... 14

5.1. Understanding the Role of Superfoods in Weight Management ... 14

5.2. Macronutrients and Weight Management ... 14

5.3. Protein ... 15

5.4. Carbohydrates ... 15

5.5. Fats ... 15

5.6. Super Greens for Weight Management ... 15

5.7. Spirulina ... 16

5.8. Kale ... 16

5.9. Weight Management with Fruits ... 16

5.10. Avocado ... 16

5.11. Berries ... 16

5.12. The Role of Nuts and Seeds ... 17

5.13. Almonds ... 17

5.14. Chia Seeds ... 17

5.15. Super Beverages for Weight Management ... 17

5.16. Green Tea ... 17

5.17. Coffee ... 17

6. Heart-Healthy Helpers: Superfoods for Cardiovascular Health ... 19

6.1. The Omega-3 All-Stars ... 19

6.2. Fiber-Rich Foods: Your Heart's Cleaning Crew ... 20

6.3. Antioxidant Powerhouses ... 20

6.4. Nuts and Seeds: The Heart-Healthy Snack ... 21

6.5. The Magic of Monounsaturated Fats ... 21

6.6. The Colourful World of Fruits and Vegetables ... 21

7. Digestive Dynamos: Superfoods for Gut Health ... 23

7.1. Understanding Your Gut 23

7.2. Why Superfoods for Gut Health? 23

7.3. Superfoods for a Healthy Gut 24

7.4. Ways to Incorporate Superfoods into Your Diet 25

7.5. Maintaining Optimal Gut Health 25

8. Mood Modulators: Superfoods for Mental Well-being 26

8.1. Nourishing the Brain: Nutrients and Their Role 26

8.2. Superfoods for Mental Well-being 27

8.3. Superfoods in Everyday Diet: Practical Tips 28

9. Endurance Enhancers: Superfoods for Energy and Stamina . . . 30

9.1. The Supercharged Power Providers 30

9.2. Harnessing the Energy Burst from Green Powerhouses . . . 31

9.3. The Sweet Energy Potions 31

9.4. The Fatigue Fighter: Hydration 32

9.5. The Energizing World of Seeds 32

9.6. Conclusion: Power Your Body Right 32

10. Age Defying Aliments: Superfoods for Longevity and Anti-
Aging 34

10.1. Pomegranates: The Ruby-Red Elixirs of Life 34

10.2. Dark Chocolate: A Sinful Pleasure that's Good for You . . 34

10.3. Berries: A Colorful Spectrum of Longevity 35

10.4. Gut-Friendly Probiotics: The Underrated Allies for
Longevity 35

10.5. The Green Gold: Leafy Vegetables 35

10.6. Mighty Almonds: Small Bite, Big Benefits 36

10.7. Green Tea: A Timeless Elixir 36

10.8. Olive Oil: A Core life-Extending Ingredient of the
Mediterranean 36

11. Elevate Your Diet: Incorporating Superfoods into Daily Meals . 38

11.1. Kickstarting with Breakfast 38

11.2. Power Packed Lunches 38

11.3. Snacks and More 39

11.4. Digestive Friendly Dinners 39

11.5. Hydrate Way to Health 40

Chapter 1. Introduction

Unleash your potential to feel better, live longer and conquer every day with renewed vigor! Welcome to "The Superfood Revolution: Nutrients to Transform Your Life," a special report curated just for you. Overflowing with insights into the world's mightiest foods, this report promises a unique journey into the revitalizing power of proper nutrition. It's far from a tedious recitation of vitamins; instead, it's a vivid exploration of nature's wonder drugs—superfoods—and how you can harness their power to transform your life! This guide is the golden key to ensuring you're not just living but thriving with the energy and vitality you deserve. So, let's take a leap into the world of nature's finest gifts, because healthy living just got exciting!

Chapter 2. Understanding Superfoods: The Basics

Superfoods may sound like they hail from another planet, but these nutrition powerhouses are readily available on our own Earth. They are foods—typically fruits, vegetables, grains, nuts, and seeds—that are rich in essential nutrients, potentially beneficial for health beyond just providing basic nutrition. However, before diving into the specifics of superfoods, let's first take a deeper look at the concept behind them.

2.1. Understanding the Superfood Concept

The concept of a 'superfood' is a relatively recent invention. While hailed as wonder foods that can boost your body to superhero levels, even professional nutritionists would point out that they are, first and foremost, simply food. Many superfoods have been a staple part of human diets for thousands of years. It is only now, with our modern understanding of nutrition and health, that we are beginning to fully appreciate their benefits.

The term 'superfood' is a marketing concept more than a scientific one. You will not find it listed in a dietetic textbook or noted down in a nutritionist's ledger. However, this does not mean it is without substance. Superfoods carry this moniker as they contain higher-than-average levels of nutrients, including vitamins, minerals, antioxidants, and more. These are foods that can provide significant beneficial effects on the body when consumed as part of a balanced, healthy diet.

2.2. Nutritional Density: A Key Aspect

The central attribute that defines whether a food is 'super' is its nutritional density. This refers to the concentration of beneficial nutrients in each bite: the higher the concentration, the higher the nutritional density. Superfoods, therefore, don't just fill you up; they give you the maximum amount of health benefits for the least amount of calories, allowing you to nourish your body efficiently and effectively.

To understand nutritional density, consider this: eating a single almond provides you with a host of benefits, from healthy fats to fiber and protein. In contrast, eating a handful of potato chips may fill you up, but it provides little nutrition. The almond, therefore, is more nutritionally dense and considered a superfood.

2.3. Superfoods: More than Vitamins and Minerals

When we discuss superfoods, we delve deeper than just vitamins and minerals. While these are crucial for our body, superfoods also excel in providing antioxidants, polyphenols, fiber, and healthy fats—components that each play their role in maintaining our health.

Antioxidants, for instance, are essential in combating free radicals, reducing inflammation and helping to prevent some diseases like cancer. Polyphenols promote heart health, boost brain function, and improve digestion, among other benefits. Fiber helps maintain a healthy gut, improve digestion, reduce cholesterol levels, and balance blood sugar levels. Healthy fats—concentrated in avocados, olive oil, and flaxseed—contribute to better brain function and help control our mood.

2.4. Staying Grounded: The 'Super' Misconception

Despite the many health benefits of these foods, it's important to bear in mind one thing: no single superfood can completely meet all our daily nutritional requirements. Health cannot be achieved just by incorporating a few superfoods into an otherwise unhealthy diet. It's necessary to maintain balance and not to consider these foods as magical pills that can automatically fix health problems.

Think of superfoods as the cherry on top of a well-balanced diet. A rainbow of fruits and vegetables, whole grains, lean proteins, and healthy fats should make up the main bulk of our dietary intake, with superfoods scattered throughout to naturally enhance our nutrient intake.

In summary, superfoods are a welcome addition to a balanced diet, their high nutrient density adding that extra 'oomph' to your meals and making them excellent tools in maintaining and improving overall health. Their powerhouse status stems from their high content of vitamins, minerals, antioxidants, polyphenols, fiber, and healthy fats. However, it's essential to remember that superfoods should complement an already healthy diet, not replace it. The magic of superfoods lies in their ability to seamlessly weave themselves into our meals, making the ordinary extraordinary. Their inclusion makes every day an opportunity to fuel our bodies optimally, and that's the kind of superpower we can all use more of.

2.5. Embracing the Superfood Journey

The world of superfoods offers a wide variety to choose from—fruits, vegetables, nuts, seeds, grains, fish, and even dark chocolate—all promising enhanced health and vitality. This guide aims to assist you on your journey of embracing superfoods, identifying the worthy candidates, breaking them down, and suggesting the best ways of incorporating them into your daily life. A world of color, flavor, variety, and health awaits you.

Chapter 3. The Antioxidant Army: Superfoods for Immunity

The human body is an intricate, finely tuned machine, battling daily with environmental contaminants, processed foods, and stressors that threaten to undermine our health. Today we begin our journey with an overview of nutrients known as antioxidants, revered troops in the defense of our health, found aplenty in superfoods.

3.1. Understanding Antioxidants

Antioxidants are compounds that neutralize harmful molecules called free radicals, unavoidable byproducts of bodily processes like digestion and environmental influences like air pollutants. An overload of free radicals can destabilize other atoms and lead to oxidative stress, contributing to chronic diseases such as heart disease, diabetes, and cancer.

Antioxidants can be synthetic; however, those found in superfoods are, overwhelming, the preferred defenders. Our bodies do produce some of these essential nutrients, but not all, thus making our diet crucial in consolidating our antioxidant army.

3.2. The Superfood Squadron

Many superfoods can boost our antioxidant intake and improve overall health. From berries and nuts to herbs and vegetables, let's peek into these nature's arsenals and their benefits.

3.2.1. Berries

An undisputed leader in the antioxidant world, berries are a treasure trove of flavonoids, anthocyanins, and various other antioxidant compounds. Blueberries, renowned for their high antioxidant content, improve memory and cognitive function. Raspberries, strawberries, acai, and goji berries, with their high amounts of vitamin C, enhance immune function and protect against cellular damage.

3.2.2. Nuts and Seeds

Concentrated sources of vitamin E, an important antioxidant, nuts and seeds are royalty amongst immunity boosters. Almonds, sunflower seeds, and flaxseeds, packed with protein, fiber, and healthy fats, aid in protecting heart health and reducing inflammation.

3.2.3. Herbs and Spices

Culinary enhancers like turmeric, ginger, and cinnamon, not only add flavor but a wealth of immunity protection. Curcumin in turmeric aids in fighting inflammation, an underlying factor of chronic diseases. Gingerol in ginger has powerful anti-cancer properties. Cinnamon, rich in polyphenols, assists in regulating blood sugar levels.

3.2.4. Leafy Greens

Spinach, kale, and chard are some of the leafy greens abundant in antioxidant vitamins like C, E, beta-carotene, and several flavonoids. They also house the crucial mineral selenium necessary for the optimal function of many antioxidant enzymes in our body.

3.3. Empower Your Diet with Antioxidant-rich Superfoods

Daily consumption of antioxidant-rich superfoods substantially contributes to great health. Here's how you can make these foods a substantial part of your diet.

3.3.1. Incorporate Berries into Your Meals

Add a touch of sweetness with berries in your breakfast cereals, yogurts, or smoothies. Berry salads and desserts can be a deliciously healthy end to any meal.

3.3.2. Pair Your Meals with Nuts and Seeds

A handfull of nuts or seeds make for healthy snacks. You can also sprinkle them over salads, stews or use them in baked goods for added texture and flavor.

3.3.3. Get Creative with Herbs and Spices

Try to incorporate herbs and spices into your recipes. Turmeric lattes, ginger teas and cinnamon-infused desserts not only boost your immunity but also add warmth and depth to your dishes.

3.3.4. Regularly Consume Leafy Greens

Include leafy greens in daily meals. They can be turned into salads, incorporated into sandwiches and wraps, added to smoothies, or sautéed as side dishes.

3.4. Beware of Excess

While antioxidants are essential, remember that balance is key.

Consuming antioxidant-rich foods in excess can have detrimental effects, possibly leading to toxicity and impaired immunity. Aim for variety, as different superfoods provide different kinds of antioxidants, and balance ensures you attract a wide spectrum of health benefits.

With the understanding and practical ways to incorporate antioxidant-rich superfoods into your diet, the path to boosting immunity is clearer. These are not just everyday ingredients; they are soldiers in your antioxidant army, rising against the onslaught of disease and paving the path towards optimal health and vitality.

The journey does not stop here. We'll continue to delve further into the world of superfoods and the wonders they can do for our bodies. After all, knowledge is power, and understanding how to fuel your body with proper nutrition is one of the highest forms of self-care. Stay tuned!

Chapter 4. Brain Power: Superfoods for Cognitive Function

Superfoods are not only capable of supporting your physical health, but they also play a significant role in boosting cognitive function. Consuming a variety of superfoods may enhance memory, focus, and other cognitive processes.

4.1. Understanding the Brain-Food Connection

The foods we consume significantly influence our overall brain health and cognitive function. Some nutrients are particularly useful for the brain. They not only provide fuel for the body, but they also create essential neurotransmitters and protect the brain from damage and aging.

Omega-3 fatty acids, for instance, are necessary for brain health. Approximately 60% of our brain is fat, and half of that fat is the omega-3 type. Omega-3s are important for brain health because they provide essential building blocks for the brain. They're also crucial for learning and memory.

The following are several superfoods that can improve cognitive function.

4.2. 1. Berries

Berries, such as strawberries, blueberries, blackberries, and raspberries, are full of antioxidants. These antioxidants may delay brain aging and enhance memory. Many berries contain flavonoids, specifically anthocyanidins, known to improve brain health.

Berries and other foods with deep pigmentation are rich in antioxidants, which help control damaging free radicals. Antioxidants also stimulate the neural pathways, improving memory and cognitive function.

4.3. 2. Fatty Fish

Fatty fish is a rich source of omega-3 fatty acids, a major building block in the brain. Omega-3s play a vital role in sharpening memory and improving mood, as well as protecting your brain against decline.

Salmon, trout, and sardines are among the fish with the largest proportional content of omega-3. Not only do these superfoods improve brain health, but they are also good for the heart.

4.4. 3. Dark Chocolate

Dark chocolate and cocoa powder are packed with a few brain-boosting compounds, including caffeine, antioxidants, and flavonoids.

Flavonoids are a group of antioxidant plant compounds that are particularly important for brain health, as they seem to help areas of the brain involved in learning and memory.

4.5. 4. Green Tea

Just like dark chocolate, green tea has caffeine and antioxidants that can enhance brain function. L-theanine, a type of amino acid in green tea, can cross the blood-brain barrier and increase the activity of the neurotransmitter GABA, which has anti-anxiety effects. It also increases dopamine and the production of alpha waves in the brain.

4.6. 5. Turmeric

This deep-yellow spice is a key ingredient in curry powder and has a number of benefits for the brain. Curcumin, the active ingredient in turmeric, has been shown to cross the blood-brain barrier. It has antioxidant and anti-inflammatory benefits that can directly enter the brain and benefit the cells there.

4.7. 6. Broccoli

Rich in antioxidants and vitamin K, broccoli is believed to support brain health. As a matter of fact, several studies link a higher vitamin K intake to better memory. Beyond vitamin K, broccoli contains a number of compounds that give it anti-inflammatory and antioxidant effects, which may help protect the brain against damage.

4.8. 7. Pumpkin Seeds

Pumpkin seeds contain powerful antioxidants that protect the body and brain from free radical damage. They're also an excellent source of magnesium, iron, zinc, and copper.

4.9. Implementing Superfoods into Your Diet

One of the most effective and simplest ways to maintain brain health is by incorporating superfoods into your diet. Here are few suggestions on how to include them into your daily routine.

1. Start your day with a smoothie. Blend together some dark leafy greens like spinach or kale with fruit such as bananas and blueberries. Add a spoonful of chia seeds or flaxseeds for an added nutrient boost.

2. Try to incorporate fish into your meals twice a week. Freshly grilled salmon with a side of steamed broccoli makes for a nutrient-packed meal.

3. When you're feeling peckish in between meals, reach for a handful of nuts like almonds or walnuts, which contain essential fats beneficial for brain health.

4. You can also sprinkle pumpkin seeds on your salad or stir them into your yogurt for an added crunch and nutrient boost.

5. Consider switching your regular cup of coffee for green tea, which not only helps with brain function but may also lower your risk of heart disease.

6. For dessert, opt for a square or two of dark chocolate. Look for chocolate with a cocoa content of 70% or higher.

4.10. A Word of Caution

While these superfoods are beneficial for brain health, they are part of a larger lifestyle that supports cognitive function. Regular exercise, plenty of sleep, not smoking, limited alcohol consumption, stress management, and mental activities all contribute to brain health.

Remember that although these superfoods can support brain health, they are not a cure for cognitive disorders or a substitute for professional medical advice or treatment. If you or a loved one experience concerning cognitive symptoms, consult a healthcare provider.

Overall, embracing a diet filled with the vibrant, nutrient-dense superfoods mentioned above can usher significant improvements in cognitive health. United with a balanced lifestyle, your journey towards better brain health can become an exciting and rewarding exploration of the delectable treasures nature has to offer.

Chapter 5. Weight Warriors: Superfoods for Weight Management

Whether you're battling the bulge, striving to maintain a healthy weight, or simply looking for more energy throughout your day, superfoods can be your secret weapon.

5.1. Understanding the Role of Superfoods in Weight Management

First and foremost, it's essential to understand what exactly makes a food 'super.' Nutritionists often use this label to describe foods that are low in calories while being high in nutrients. They're also packed with vitamins, minerals, and antioxidants — compounds that help your body function at its peak. Consuming these superfoods can not only assist your body in operating more efficiently but specifically aid in weight management.

5.2. Macronutrients and Weight Management

The three primary macronutrients our bodies require are proteins, carbohydrates, and fats. Each serves a unique purpose, and while they're all necessary for our bodies to function correctly, not all sources are created equal when it comes to weight management. Let's take a deeper look.

5.3. Protein

Protein assists with weight management by increasing satiety—the feeling of fullness—and reducing hunger. We should prioritize lean sources of protein, like fish, chicken, plant-based proteins (beans, lentils, chickpeas), tocopherols, Greek yogurt, and eggs.

5.4. Carbohydrates

Contrary to popular belief, carbs are not your enemy. However, choosing the right types—complex carbohydrates—is essential. These good carbs are digested slower and offer more sustainable energy, eliminating the spikes in blood sugar associated with simple carbohydrates. Superfoods rich in complex carbs include whole grains, such as oats and brown rice, and vegetables like sweet potatoes and butternut squash.

5.5. Fats

A healthy diet includes the right types of fats, namely monounsaturated and polyunsaturated fats. These healthy fats can help reduce bad cholesterol levels, increasing heart health. Avocados, salmon, nuts and seeds, and olive oil are great sources of these beneficial fats.

5.6. Super Greens for Weight Management

Super green foods are nutritional powerhouses that provide immense health benefits due to their antioxidant, fiber, and phytonutrient content. Known for their high vitamin and mineral content, consuming these superfoods can result in boosted energy, enhanced detoxification, and improved digestion, all contributing to weight management.

5.7. Spirulina

This blue-green algae is a protein-rich superfood packed with vitamins B1, B2, and B3, iron, magnesium, and potassium. It is also low in calories, making it a perfect aid for weight control.

5.8. Kale

Kale helps in weight management by being a low-calorie, high-fiber superfood. It is packed with vitamins A, K, and C and is an excellent source of calcium and iron.

5.9. Weight Management with Fruits

But it isn't all just about green veggies and proteins. Certain fruits are also packed with fiber and other key nutrients that help control hunger, promote fullness, and prevent overeating.

5.10. Avocado

High in monounsaturated fats, avocado aids in weight management by promoting a feeling of fullness and reducing the urge to overeat. Moreover, it is a great source of fiber and protein.

5.11. Berries

Berries like blueberries, strawberries, and raspberries are rich in fiber, which slows down digestion and makes you feel fuller for longer—thus helping to manage weight.

5.12. The Role of Nuts and Seeds

Nuts and seeds might be small, but they're mighty when it comes to weight management. They pack a punch of protein, fiber, and healthy fats, promoting fullness and warding off hunger.

5.13. Almonds

Almonds are high in protein, fiber, and monounsaturated fats. A handful of these crunchy delights can help curb your appetite and prevent overeating.

5.14. Chia Seeds

Chia seeds are rich in fiber and can absorb large quantities of water, expanding in your stomach and reducing hunger.

5.15. Super Beverages for Weight Management

The drinks we consume can play a significant role in our weight management efforts. Several superfood beverages can support weight loss and maintenance due to their nutrient compositions.

5.16. Green Tea

Rich in antioxidants and other plant compounds, green tea has been associated with increased fat burning and weight loss.

5.17. Coffee

Coffee can boost your metabolism and help you burn more calories, primarily due to its caffeine content.

Hopefully, this comprehensive guide provides you with an understanding of how particular superfoods can aid in weight management. Remember, it's not just about dropping pounds—it's about nourishing your body with the right nutrients to function optimally. Make these superfoods a part of your diet, and watch them work their magic!

Chapter 6. Heart-Healthy Helpers: Superfoods for Cardiovascular Health

Perhaps there's no organ that receives as much emphasis as the heart when referring to health. And rightly so; it is the engine that powers every aspect of our being, tirelessly circulating oxygen and nutrients through a network of veins and arteries. But what fuels the heart? Here, we navigate the fascinating influence of superfoods on cardiovascular health, charting a course that'll lead to longevity and vitality.

While the advent of modern medicine has brought forth a myriad of advancements, the ancient proverb still rings true: "An ounce of prevention is worth a pound of cure." Thus, the first step towards a heart-healthy lifestyle lies in nutrition. The importance of diet cannot be overstressed. But don't consider this as a restriction; envision it as an opportunity to introduce a bountiful assortment of delicious, heart-boosting superfoods into your daily meals.

6.1. The Omega-3 All-Stars

Omega-3 fatty acids represent the superstars of heart-healthy nutrients. Research tirelessly attests to their ability in lowering heart rate and blood pressure, reducing the risk of abnormal heart rhythm, and lessening the probability of sudden cardiac death. Boasting potent anti-inflammatory properties, Omega-3 fatty acids also help keep blood vessels healthy.

Prominent among these life-saving wonders are cold-water fish like salmon, mackerel, sardines, and tuna. Yet, as power-packed as these sources are, they're not the only vehicles for Omega-3. For those wishing to avoid animal products, alternatives abound. Chia seeds, flaxseeds, hemp seeds, Walnuts, and even vegetables like Brussels sprouts also carry substantial amounts of this essential nutrient.

6.2. Fiber-Rich Foods: Your Heart's Cleaning Crew

Like diligent janitors, fiber-rich foods do an excellent job of cleaning up after meals. Soluble fiber acts like a sponge; it soaks up the "bad" cholesterol, preventing it from clogging arteries and leading to heart disease. Foods notably high in soluble fiber include oatmeal, barley, beans, lentils, fruits like apples and berries, and vegetables such as okra and eggplant.

In addition, regular consumption of these naturally nutrient-dense foods can help you maintain a healthy weight—a critical factor for preventing heart disease.

6.3. Antioxidant Powerhouses

We often hear of antioxidants, but what exactly are these vital substances? Antioxidants are compounds that neutralize harmful free radicals within our bodies, which can lead to cell damage and chronic disease, including heart disease. This makes them an essential ally in our journey towards heart-friendly nutrition.

Berries are an incredibly potent source of antioxidants, carrying massive amounts of anthocyanins, vitamin C and fiber. Other antioxidant-rich superfoods include dark chocolate, cherries, artichokes, kidney beans, and pecans. Moreover, leafy greens like spinach and kale are full of heart-promoting properties, with valuable antioxidants like lutein, beta-carotene, and vitamin C.

6.4. Nuts and Seeds: The Heart-Healthy Snack

Nuts and seeds reign supreme amongst heart-healthy snacks. Almonds, walnuts, pistachios, chia seeds, and flaxseeds are cuddling a treasure trove of beneficial nutrients like healthy fats, fiber, and antioxidants. Evidence is strong for their role in reducing heart disease risk factors, and encouraging regular, moderate intake.

Nuts and seeds are quite versatile too. Add them to smoothies for an added crunch, or enjoy a handful as an afternoon snack. So, the next time you feel puckish, skip the chips and dip into a nourishing bag of nuts or seeds instead.

6.5. The Magic of Monounsaturated Fats

Monounsaturated fats improve the body's levels of 'bad' LDL cholesterol and increase 'good' HDL cholesterol. Foods rich in these fats include avocados, olives, and most nuts and seeds, which work in concert to reduce the risk of heart disease.

6.6. The Colourful World of Fruits and Vegetables

Fruits and vegetables are not to be sidelined in our cardiovascular health journey. Their vibrant hues are indicative of the diverse range of health-boosting nutrients they carry. From beta-carotene in carrots, lycopene in tomatoes to resveratrol in red grapes, these vital substances lower the chances of heart disease and stroke. Aim for at least five portions of a variety of fruits and veggies each day for the best results.

While it can be a challenge to overhaul your eating habits, it certainly isn't impossible. Remember, the key to a successful diet is balance. Encourage diversity and moderation in your food selection. Make conscious decisions to choose foods that nourish and boost your heart health. Your choice to embrace these superfoods not only sets the stage for a more vibrant life but also marks a decisive step towards lifelong wellness. Embrace this splendid superfood revolution today, because your heart deserves nothing less!

Chapter 7. Digestive Dynamos: Superfoods for Gut Health

In the realm of bodily functions, digestion holds the key to a happier and healthier you. Held within the intricate labyrinth of your gut are billions of bacteria working round the clock. They break down the food you eat, absorb the necessary nutrients, and fuel your body's overall functioning. So, maintaining optimal gut health should sit atop your wellness checklist. Superfoods can assist, infusing your system with essential nutrients that promote a harmonious symbiosis between you and your gut flora. Let's dive deeper.

7.1. Understanding Your Gut

Your gut (gastrointestinal tract) is more than a simple pathway for food, spanning from your mouth to your anus. It's a bustling microcosm, with over 100 trillion microbes, collectively known as gut flora or gut microbiota. These include bacteria, viruses, and fungi whose chief job is to break down food into absorbable nutrients.

The gut microbiota influences your health in multiple ways. It aids in food digestion, supports immune function, balances your metabolism, and even impacts your mood. An unhealthy gut, marked by an imbalance in the microbiota, might lead to issues such as weight gain, high blood sugar, stomach discomfort, and more. Cue superfoods, which can help maintain a healthy gut biodiversity.

7.2. Why Superfoods for Gut Health?

Superfoods for gut health are high in fiber, which serves as fuel for your gut bacteria, helping in their multiplication and diversity.

They're also rich in polyphenols (plant compounds with antioxidative properties) and essential vitamins, like vitamin C and K, that provide a wide array of health benefits.

Diets abundant in superfoods lead to a proliferating gut microbiota, yielding short-chain fatty acids (SCFAs). These SCFAs play a crucial role in maintaining gut health. They nourish the gut lining, ensuring optimal absorption of nutrients while simultaneously maintaining an effective barrier against harmful substances.

7.3. Superfoods for a Healthy Gut

- **Garlic:** High in inulin, a type of prebiotic fiber, garlic is a potent detoxifying agent that helps strengthen the gut flora, providing relief from various digestive issues. It also contains a compound, allicin, associated with anticancer, antioxidant, antibacterial, and anti-inflammatory effects.

- **Kimchi:** This fermented Korean dish, teeming with probiotics, is an outstanding choice for gut health. It's made from cabbage, radish, or cucumber mixed with chili pepper, garlic, and other spices. The dish offers fiber and rich amounts of vitamins A, B, and C.

- **Chia seeds:** Rich in fiber and Omega-3 fatty acids, chia seeds expand in the stomach, promoting fullness and slow absorption of food. This reduces the chances of blood sugar spikes and supports the growth of beneficial gut bacteria.

- **Beetroot:** Brimming with dietary fiber, betalains, folate, and vitamin C, beetroot promotes digestion and helps maintain steady bowel movements. It is also known to assist in liver detoxification.

- **Bananas:** Mild and easy to digest, bananas are excellent for restoring health to your gut. They are rich in fiber and contain a type of carbohydrate called pectin, which assists in the removal of heavy metals and toxins from the body.

7.4. Ways to Incorporate Superfoods into Your Diet

Incorporating these superfoods in your diet isn't difficult. You could start your day with a delicious smoothie made from bananas, chia seeds, and a variety of berries. For lunch and dinner, include abundant portions of leafy greens and lean proteins along with fermented foods like kimchi. Add chopped fresh garlic to your dishes for extra flavor, and end your day with a soothing drink made from fresh turmeric and ginger.

Remember to be patient; gut health improvement isn't an overnight process. Aim for consistent, healthy eating habits instead of quick fixes.

7.5. Maintaining Optimal Gut Health

While incorporating these superfoods in your diet is essential, maintaining a healthy lifestyle is just as important. Regular exercise, adequate sleep, stress management, and limited alcohol intake can all contribute to improved gut health.

Research into gut health is evolving, with new insights emerging regularly. As scientists continue to unravel the gut's intricacies, one thing remains clear: taking care of your gut microbiota is a giant stride towards overall well-being. Armed with knowledge and the right superfoods, you're well equipped to enhance your gut health, paving the way for a healthier, more vibrant life.

Chapter 8. Mood Modulators: Superfoods for Mental Well-being

Hidden within nature's bounty lies a plethora of edibles with the power to enhance our mood and uplift our spirits. As science delves deeper into understanding how food impacts our mental well-being, we unearth an increasing number of mood modulating superfoods packed with essential nutrients that act as fuel for our brain. This chapter uncovers some of these natural miracle workers, offering insights into how they foster mental wellness.

8.1. Nourishing the Brain: Nutrients and Their Role

Every snack we consume, every sip we take, influences the intricate interplay of hormones, neurotransmitters, and metabolic processes in our bodies. The brain, akin to a high-functioning engine, requires premium-grade fuel to thrive. The fuel, in this instance, is a balanced diet replete with mood-enhancing nutrients.

To better comprehend how our dietary choices influence our mood, we must first understand the nutritional elements pertinent to brain health.

Omega-3 Fatty Acids: Omega-3 fatty acids are fundamental building blocks of the brain. These fats aid in constructing cell membranes, fostering neuron function, and reducing inflammation. Deficiency of Omega-3 acids may amplify risks of mood disorders. Foods rich in Omega-3s include fatty fish, walnuts, and chia seeds.

Tryptophan: Tryptophan, an essential amino acid, is a precursor to serotonin, a neurotransmitter popularly known as the 'happy chemical.' Serotonin contributes significantly to happiness and well-being. You can find tryptophan in foods like turkey, eggs, cheese, and Pineapples.

B-Vitamins: Certain vitamins, particularly B-Vitamins including B6, B9 (folic acid), and B12, participate in the synthesis of brain chemicals that regulate mood. Prolonged deficiency can potentially induce depression. You can find these B-vitamins in leafy greens, legumes, citrus fruits, and lean meats.

8.2. Superfoods for Mental Well-being

Using the blueprint of brain-boosting nutrients, let's traverse the spectrum of superfoods that are your best allies for mental well-being.

Berries: Bursting with antioxidants, berries confront oxidative stress and inflammation, which are invariably implicated in mood disorders. Berries are rich in anthocyanidins that cross the blood-brain barrier, supporting brain health. Add a serving of berries in your daily diet to uplift your mood.

Leafy Greens: Kale, spinach, and other leafy greens are powerhouses of mental wellness nutrients. In particular, they are abundant in folate, whose deficiency is linked to depressive symptoms. The punch of antioxidants that accompany these greens offers further mood-uplifting benefits.

Fermented Foods: Fermented foods like yogurt, kimchi and miso are probiotic-rich, thereby promoting a healthy gut microbiome. Noteworthy, gut health remarkably influences mental well-being owing to the gut-brain axis; a healthy gut can, hence, lead to a happy mind.

Oily Fish: A rich source of DHA, a type of Omega-3 fatty acid, oily fish like salmon, mackerel, and trout can keep mood disorders at bay by supporting brain function and reducing inflammation.

Cacao: Dark chocolate, specifically, is rich in flavonoids, caffeine, and theobromine - mood enhancing substances that double up to also reduce depression and improve brain function.

8.3. Superfoods in Everyday Diet: Practical Tips

How can we integrate these mood-enhancing superfoods into our daily eating habits, you ask? Here are some practical tips:

1. **Make a Rainbow Plate**: Add as many colorful veggies and fruits to your meal as possible. Besides offering a delightful visual, it'll ensure that you're receiving an array of different nutrients.

2. **Mindful Snacking**: Instead of succumbing to unhealthy processed snacks during those mid-day hunger pangs, opt for nuts, seeds or berries.

3. **Hydrate**: Dehydration can make you feel lethargic and negatively impact mood. So make it a habit to drink ample water throughout the day.

4. **Opt for Whole Foods**: As far as possible, choose whole, unprocessed foods as they contain more nutrients and fewer artificial additives.

In weaving a narrative around food and mood, it's crucial to remember that a 'one size fits all' approach doesn't apply. Individual nutritional needs and responses vary. Hence, while these superfoods are established for their mental well-being benefits, the key lies in aligning them with your personal nutritional requirements.

In concluding, shifting your diet to incorporate these superfoods can work wonders in uplifting your spirits and fostering mental wellness. Remember, your state of mind isn't solely a manifestation of thoughts and experiences, but also the nutrients that you feed your brain!

Chapter 9. Endurance Enhancers: Superfoods for Energy and Stamina

Every step towards better health starts with one profound concept — energy is EVERYTHING. Energy fuels our brain, commands our muscles, and provides sustenance to every cell in our bodies. Just like a car that runs on gas, our bodies require good quality fuel, that energy, to function optimally. This fuel comes from the food we eat and the beverages we drink, making it crucial to choose wisefully to live fully.

9.1. The Supercharged Power Providers

When you need an energy boost, it is tempting to reach for energy drinks or a quick hit of caffeine. While these may induce a quick burst of energy, they often lead to a sudden 'crash'. Superfoods are energy-boosting alternatives that release energy slowly and constantly over time, helping to maintain steady energy levels throughout the day.

Legumes such as lentils are high in fiber and complex carbohydrates. This means they are digested slowly, giving a continuous supply of energy. Lentils are also rich in folate, iron, and manganese, which play a significant role in energy production and circulation.

Nuts, such as almonds, have a healthful mix of protein, fiber, and healthy fats, making them an excellent source of sustained energy. They're also packed with vitamins and minerals essential for energy production, including B vitamins, magnesium, and iron.

Quinoa is a grain that's high in proteins, fiber, and complex carbohydrates. It is also one of the few plant-based foods that contain all the essential amino acids. Eating quinoa helps maintain steady blood sugar levels, thus providing lasting energy.

9.2. Harnessing the Energy Burst from Green Powerhouses

Green superfoods, namely, spinach, kale, and broccoli, should be your go-to for enhancing endurance. Why? These leafy greens are rich in iron, a mineral key to the production of hemoglobin that aids in oxygen transportation to the muscles, boosting energy and endurance.

Spirulina, a blue-green algae, is a nutritional powerhouse that provides a quick energy boost due to its richness in proteins, Vitamins B1, B2, and B3, copper, iron, alongside other essential minerals. Being easily digestible as well, it provides an instant energy surge without straining your digestive system.

9.3. The Sweet Energy Potions

For those with a sweet tooth, nature lends a helping hand through fruits. Bananas are power-packed with natural sugars, fiber, and potassium, providing a quick, substantial energy boost. Berries, rich in fiber and antioxidants, release energy slowly keeping you powered up for longer.

Further, avocados are not just a fit-foodie favorite for nothing. They contain high-quality fats (mono and polyunsaturated fats), fibers, and vitamins, making them a perfect energy-stimulating snack.

9.4. The Fatigue Fighter: Hydration

Staying hydrated serves as one of the simplest ways to keep our energy levels up. Dehydration can lead to fatigue as it impacts the volume of blood pumped by the heart. Therefore, drinking enough water and hydrating beverages is instrumental in maintaining energy levels.

Coconut water serves as nature's Gatorade. It is a great source of several vital minerals like potassium, magnesium, sodium, and calcium which contribute to hydration and recovery, particularly for physically active individuals.

9.5. The Energizing World of Seeds

Seeds of diverse varieties have made it to the superfood club, primarily chia seeds and flax seeds. Chia seeds have an impressive nutritional profile rich in fiber, protein, healthy omega-3 fats, and a host of micronutrients that help maintain high energy levels.

Flaxseeds, on the other hand, are a potent source of the omega-3 fatty acids, protein, and fiber. There's also an additional benefit: lignans. These plant compounds possess antioxidant properties, adding an additional energy-boosting edge.

9.6. Conclusion: Power Your Body Right

Boosting endurance isn't about quick fixes. It's about a sustained, conscious effort to fuel the body right and keep your energy levels stoked throughout the day. Reach for these endurance-enhancing superfoods and let your energy and stamina skyrocket. Plus, remember to stay hydrated, honor your need for rest, and finally, consult your healthcare provider when implementing any new nutrition strategies.

Remember, you aren't what you eat; you're what you absorb, so take your time, eat slowly, savor each bite, and be present. Treat your body like the spectacular, energy crafting machine it is, feed it with the finest, and watch your life transform, one energized day at a time.

Chapter 10. Age Defying Aliments: Superfoods for Longevity and Anti-Aging

Longevity and anti-aging, once the province of fables and myths, are slowly becoming tangible goals due to the advancements in modern medical science, healthy lifestyle choices, and the power of superfoods. With their potent and unique combination of crucial vitamins, minerals, and antioxidants, these superfoods possess an extraordinary capacity to mitigate the effects of aging and prolong our lifespan.

10.1. Pomegranates: The Ruby-Red Elixirs of Life

Pomegranates, ancient fruits that have been revered in various cultures for millennia, are a fountain of youth. Packed with an abundant supply of antioxidants like punicalagins and punicic acid, pomegranates combat aging by minimizing free-radical damage, which accelerates aging. They also foster heart health, reducing the risk of cardiovascular diseases—one of the biggest threats to longevity today.

10.2. Dark Chocolate: A Sinful Pleasure that's Good for You

Much to the delight of chocolate lovers, dark chocolate is a superfood packed with anti-aging benefits. Rich in flavanols and antioxidants, it works to improve skin elasticity, reduce inflammation, decrease 'bad' LDL cholesterol, and equip the body to combat free radical damage. The key to unlocking these benefits lies in choosing dark chocolate with a high cocoa content and consuming it in moderation.

10.3. Berries: A Colorful Spectrum of Longevity

Blueberries, strawberries, raspberries, and blackberries—these humble garden fruits are powerhouses of antioxidant activity. Packed with vitamins, fiber and particularly powerful compounds called anthocyanins, berries are known to delay brain aging and enhance memory, battle off heart diseases, and even combat cancer.

10.4. Gut-Friendly Probiotics: The Underrated Allies for Longevity

Probiotics—found in yogurt, kefir, and fermented foods like kimchi and sauerkraut—are not as often associated with longevity as they should be. However, these bacteria are valuable health promoters that aid digestion, strengthen the immune system, and even improve mental health. Apart from these benefits, probiotics are speculated to slow aging by reducing inflammation and oxidative stress.

10.5. The Green Gold: Leafy Vegetables

Consuming a variety of leafy greens, such as kale, spinach, and collards, can significantly contribute to longevity and vitality. High in vitamins A, C, E, and K, and packed with fiber, leafy vegetables keep your heart healthy, sharpen your mind, and help your body fend off cancer. Moreover, lutein and beta-carotene, found in these green gifts from nature, keep your eyes healthy as you age.

10.6. Mighty Almonds: Small Bite, Big Benefits

Almonds are among the most nutrient-dense foods, providing a generous dose of antioxidants, vitamin E, fiber and healthy fats. Regular consumption of almonds and almond oil can help to boost heart health, maintain healthy skin, lower cholesterol levels, and help in weight management; all of which contribute to longevity.

10.7. Green Tea: A Timeless Elixir

For centuries, green tea has been an integral part of East Asia's health and longevity secret. It is rich in polyphenols, which have effects like reducing inflammation and helping fight cancer. Epigallocatechin-3-gallate (EGCG), a compound present in green tea, is another powerful compound that inhibits cell damage, fostering longevity.

10.8. Olive Oil: A Core life-Extending Ingredient of the Mediterranean

One standout food in the reported longevity of people living in the Mediterranean region is olive oil. Rich in monounsaturated fats and powerful antioxidants known as polyphenols, olive oil features anti-inflammatory properties, protects against heart disease, and combats neurodegenerative disease.

Every one of these superfoods possesses its unique way of stalling the aging process, offering additional health benefits as a bonus. It's recommended to incorporate a variety of these anti-aging, longevity-promoting superfoods into your daily meals.

Now, remember, while it is important to note the effect of superfoods on lifespan, it's equally crucial to remember that superfoods alone cannot do wonders. A sedentary lifestyle filled with stress and harmful habits like smoking and excess alcohol will indeed negate their positive effects. That being said, the diligent inclusion of these nutrient-dense superfoods into your diet, combined with regular exercise, stress management, and a positive outlook on life, might truly be the elixir of youth humans have sought since the dawn of time.

Chapter 11. Elevate Your Diet: Incorporating Superfoods into Daily Meals

Elevating your diet with the inclusion of superfoods need not be a challenging task. By understanding the importance of these foods and incorporating them creatively into your daily meals, you will initiate a transformative chapter in your life journey. Stacked high with essential nutrients, superfoods hold the keys to boosting immune function, reducing inflammation, warding off chronic diseases, and heightening overall wellness—the staple elements for nurturing a healthier, happier, and longer life.

11.1. Kickstarting with Breakfast

Begin each day by flooding your body with nourishment. Including superfoods in your breakfast can set the tone for your day, ensuring you start with an energy-packed, nutrient dense meal.

Breakfast porridge can become a nutrient powerhouse when topped with superfood fruits like blueberries, which are abundant in antioxidants. Throw in a handful of walnuts or flaxseeds for another layer of nutrients and a burst of crunchiness. Known for their high concentrations of Omega-3 fatty acids, these tiny ingredients protect heart health and support cognitive function. Moreover, a dollop of nutrient-dense Greek yogurt can uplift your calcium and protein intake—an essential fuel for your muscles and bones.

11.2. Power Packed Lunches

Concocting a nutrient-dense lunch goes beyond mere salads filled with leafy greens—although they are a formidable fortress of fiber.

It's about choosing superfood ingredients that boost nutritional value.

Quinoa, a complete protein grain, could replace your usual side of white rice. Rich in essential amino acids, it is considered a fantastic plant-based protein source. Mix in raw or lightly sautéed veggies like broccoli, kale, or spinach—each packed with powerful antioxidants and dietary fiber. A side of grilled salmon—brimming with Omega-3s—strengthens the balance of proteins.

A dressing of extra virgin olive oil, known for its heart-health benefits, paired with a dash of lemon for vitamin C uplifts the flavor profiles. A garnish of sunflower seeds or pumpkin seeds can round off the meal, contributing a welcome crunch and a punch of essential minerals and vitamins.

11.3. Snacks and More

Snacking can become a convenience-oriented downfall of many health-minded individuals. Processed snacks, crisps, or sugary confectioneries appear a tempting option when hunger strikes, but superfood alternatives exist, promising a tasty, nutritious respite.

Instead, consider a serving of almonds, renowned for their heart-healthy fats and vitamin E content. Combine these with dried goji berries—an antioxidant powerhouse—and you have a snack treat that's both satisfying and health-conscious. Or, for an energy-boosting quick-fix, dabble in a smoothie with the superfood of the superfruits—avocado. Famed for its healthy fats and fiber, pairing this creamy delight with a banana or a handful of spinach makes for a revitalizing midday snack.

11.4. Digestive Friendly Dinners

Dinner needs to meet the dual objectives—comforting after a long day, and healthful to aid proper digestion and sleep. Lentils, chickpeas, or black beans provide a protein-packed basis for many dinner dishes and are high in fiber, vital for healthy gut function. Single clove garlic—a lesser-known superfood with potent antibacterial properties—can add a flavorful punch to your dinners.

Choose lean protein like chicken or turkey, and serve alongside a salad made of mixed greens, cherry tomatoes, and cucumber. A dessert of dark chocolate, exceptionally high in antioxidants, can curb sweet tooth cravings while offering heart-health benefits.

11.5. Hydrate Way to Health

Often, we forget that hydration is a key aspect of health. Opting for superfood-infused beverages can play a substantial role in maintaining overall vitality.

Green tea—a superfood in its own right—offers catechins, potent antioxidants with proven health benefits. Lemon water kick-starts the metabolism, while a smoothie of Greek yogurt, strawberries, blueberries, and a spoonful of honey provides an energy-zapped body with a refreshing pick-me-up.

To elevate your standard hydration, consider coconut water. Blessed with electrolytes and deliciously hydrating, it's a superior substitute for sugar-loaded sports drinks, replenishing your body naturally.

In conclusion, the key to incorporating superfoods into your daily meals lies in imagination, experimentation, and understanding their health benefits. By swapping out the mundane with nutrient-dense superfoods, not only are we creating an exciting, flavorful journey for our palates, but also actively boosting our health and well-being. Every mealtime, every snack, every beverage provides a distinct opportunity to fuel the body with what it truly deserves—superior nutrition for superior health.

www.ingramcontent.com/pod-product-compliance
Lightning Source LLC
Chambersburg PA
CBHW071038260726
48661CB00007B/3052